elementary
weight loss

Elementary Weight Loss

A SIMPLE GUIDE TO LOSING WEIGHT AND LIVING HEALTHY

Jonathan Spillman

elementary
Weight loss

The subject matter, research and ideas presented by the author within this book are not intended to take the place of advice from a trained medical professional. Before altering your diet or level of physical activity, please consult your personal physician or another qualified health professional. Both the author and the publisher of this book disclaim responsibility for the direct or indirect adverse effects resulting from following the information contained within.

Mention of specific companies and organizations in this book does not imply endorsement by the author or publisher, nor does it mean specific companies and organizations endorse this book, the author or publisher. Internet addresses and related information given in this book were accurate at the time of publication.

Dedicated to Coach Bennett, who was the first person to truly provide me with the capability and motivation to lose weight.

"If you can't explain it to a six year old,
you don't understand it yourself."
- Albert Einstein

Table of Contents

Introduction

I n the summer of 2005, I tipped the scale at 282 pounds. As I stood there in silence, I couldn't help being taunted by those big, bold numbers glaring up at me from below. I was at a true crossroads in life, and I knew if I did not make some significant changes, my record weight was certain to climb.

As a shot putter in college, being large was part of my job. Even though my workout routines during those four years were relatively consistent, I was forced to maintain a diet and weight that would by no means be incorporated within a healthy lifestyle. Upon graduation, as I ended my athletic career, I had to figure out how to transform my dieting and exercise habits to avoid heading down the path of least resistance—

massive weight gain. I was determined to make major changes to my lifestyle, but wasn't exactly sure how.

I started researching some of the popular weight loss and dieting strategies on the market, but quickly became bored and frustrated with what they had to offer. The books I read were annoyingly long for the content contained within them, and there were way too many useless rules to follow as part of each weight loss plan.

Lying in bed tossing and turning one night, it struck me that losing weight shouldn't be this complicated—but rather a simple process that I could be successful with on my own terms. As my eyes adjusted to the fluorescent light beaming from the lamp I had turned on late that night, I quickly jotted down four simple words in the notebook sitting on my nightstand—**eat less**, **exercise more**. Why shouldn't it just be that simple, I thought? Over the next six months, following a common sense approach at the heart of those four simple words, I lost 85 pounds, or about one-third of my body weight. My successful experience losing weight and continuing to live a healthy life is the basis of Elementary Weight Loss.

Our World Today

I'm sure you are familiar with the terms **overweight** and **obese**. For definitional clarity, so that we are on the same page, a person that is overweight or obese means that he or she has an abnormal or excessive amount of fat accumulation that may impair his or her health.

As of the publication of this book (according to the World Health Organization), worldwide obesity has more than doubled since 1980.

More than 1.9 billion adults 18 years and older (39%) are overweight, and of those, over 600 million (13%) are obese. Additionally, 41 million children under the age of 5 are now considered overweight or obese.

Each year, we collectively spend billions of dollars trying to drop the extra weight we carry around, and unfortunately, most of us fail. In the U.S. alone, the weight loss industry brings in more than $50 billion annually (according to Marketdata Enterprises). Many of us dabble in fad diets, appetite-suppressing pills, and meaningless exercise devices, hoping that each avenue we take will be easier than the last in producing the end results we crave—to successfully lose weight.

Numerous studies have shown that a significant portion of us that try weight loss programs fail at the very beginning, or end up eventually regaining any weight that we actually do lose. According to Gary Foster, Ph.D., clinical director of the Weight and Eating Disorders Program at the University of Pennsylvania, nearly 65% of dieters return to their pre-dieting weight within three years.

Back to Basics

Although elementary school might be best remembered as a breeding ground for cooties, the birthplace of wedgies, an excuse for naptime in the middle of the day, and a training camp for dodgeball, its actual purpose is to serve as a crucial developmental period in our lives. Elementary school is a time when the concepts of reading, writing, and arithmetic are established and begin to take shape in our minds. Our time in elementary school ultimately provides us with the basic skills that we as adults use every day in our personal and professional lives.

However, as we grow older, and in theory wiser, we sometimes take for granted the basic skills we developed as children. We lose sight of the fact that the decisions we make regarding our careers, our relationships, our health, and almost every other aspect of our daily lives are defined by fundamental and simple concepts. When we are not achieving the level of success that we desire in one area or another (e.g., our health and being overweight), it becomes essential to take a step backward and redefine certain basic skills that will help to get our lives back on the right track.

A Simple Guide
In spite of all the noise in our world today, it is possible to lose weight and keep the pounds off. True weight loss is achieved by instilling simple habits and redefining basic skills throughout multiple aspects of your daily life. Following complex meal plans, difficult workouts routines, and unconventional methods to lose weight is a waste of time and effort—and will ultimately set you up for failure in living a sustainably healthy lifestyle.

Elementary Weight Loss is a simple guide to losing weight and living a healthy life that rises above the endless variety of regimented eating and exercise schedules employed through most weight loss plans. Rather than leading you into fad diet abyss, Elementary Weight Loss gets back to the foundation of losing weight with one simple formula:

Eating Less + Exercising More = Healthy Weight Loss

As with any equation, it's important that the variables contained within are properly defined: **Eating Less** refers to eating a smaller quantity of food as well as eating fewer unhealthy foods. **Exercising More** signifies a greater frequency of exercising.

To tie everything together, the word **Elementary** is part of an easy to remember wordplay created from those four simple words I put in place when I first started losing weight. That is, the first four letters in Elementary ("ELEM") coincide with the first letters in each of the words **E**at **L**ess, **E**xercise **M**ore.

This book is composed of three core sections, each carrying an equal level of importance. The first, **Prepare for Weight Loss Success**, defines mind-set methodologies that are essential in successfully losing weight. The second, **Eat Less**, and third, **Exercise More**, provide a greater level of detail and specific strategies surrounding the concepts of eating less and exercising more.

It's important that you implement and adhere to the guidelines and strategies in each section at your own discretion, and it's up to you to figure out what works best. As long as you follow the defining principles of Elementary Weight Loss— eat less, exercise more—there is no doubt that you will be headed down the path of successfully losing weight and living healthy!

Keep It Simple and Elementary...
Eat Less, Exercise More!

prepare for weight loss success

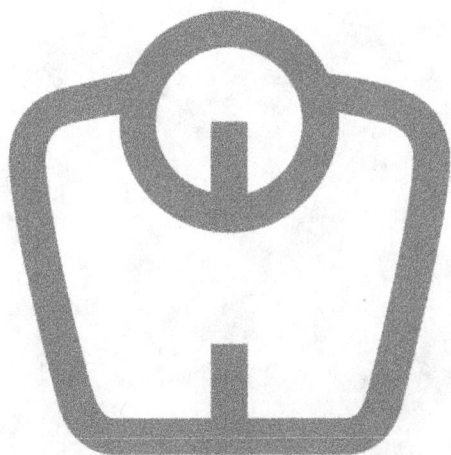

Prepare for Weight Loss Success

Growing up, I never received a normal allowance. Instead, my parents rewarded me with a certain amount of cash for every "A" I earned on school report cards, and half that amount for every "B" earned. Anything below a "B" paid nothing at all (rightfully so). In order to have any money in my wallet to spend on trading cards and action figures, I had to make sure that my grades were top notch. Money was my main motivation for succeeding in school at first, but as I grew older, attending college and leading a successful life became the primary reasons to get good grades and flourish in my studies.

My parents gave me an unbelievable amount of support and guidance growing up, teaching me to set goals and constantly work my hardest toward achieving them. I understood that in order to get accepted into a great college and be successful later in life, I would have to succeed in school. Motivation is important in any aspect of your life you hope to succeed in—especially in losing weight.

Motivation

Motivation is the key to losing weight and living healthy. Without motivation, your quest to lose weight can easily lead to failure.

To succeed, you have to have a reason and a purpose for losing weight.

Your reason and purpose will serve as a driving force of motivation throughout the weight loss process and is absolutely necessary to achieve success. Before you start your weight loss journey, ask "why" you are trying to lose weight and the real reasons you want to shed the pounds.

- Is it to improve your health?
- Is it for your spouse or significant other?

- Is it for your job and livelihood?
- Is it to improve your self-confidence?

Whatever the reasons are, don't forget why you are doing it!

Set a Weight Loss Goal

As soon as you understand why you want to lose weight, set a Weight Loss Goal (**WLG**). Choose a realistic WLG that includes the following:

- The number of pounds you want to lose.
- The ideal weight you would like to be at.
- The date by which you plan to reach your ideal weight.

It's important to set a goal that is both sensible and achievable.

Picture Yourself

According to a survey sponsored by Herbalife (conducted by Synovate eNation in 2010), one in every three overweight individuals is primarily motivated to lose weight by his or her physical appearance. That means over 600 million people around the world get motivated to lose weight just by looking in the mirror or staring at a picture of themselves.

After you set your WLG, grab a current picture of yourself. This is your **before picture**. Take a permanent marker and write in big, bold numbers across the front of the picture the number of pounds you want to lose from your WLG. Place this picture somewhere where it will get maximum visibility (e.g., on the fridge, on a nightstand, on your desk, on the dash of your car). Another (digital) option is to take a selfie on your phone, use a free photo editing tool to add the number of pounds you want to lose from your WLG, and set your before picture as the background on your phone or computer.

Your WLG posted on your before picture will be an invaluable source of motivation during the weight loss process.

Look at the picture as much as possible and have your WLG ingrained in your memory. More important, when you look at the picture, imagine yourself at your target weight—visualize the new, healthier you!

Track Progress

Progress during your weight loss journey is not just determined on the scale. Taking measurements of certain areas of your body, noting changes in the size of your clothes, and simply seeing a physical difference in your appearance are all important in tracking your weight loss progress. Whether it's on a spreadsheet or on a Post-it note, track your progress consistently (weekly is a good timeframe to benchmark your progress).

The Scale is Not Your Best Friend

As tempting as it might be, don't visit the scale every day. Treat it more as an acquaintance than as your best friend. This means visiting the scale only once a week. For a number of reasons, your body weight fluctuates each day.

If you measure your weight each day, you might not see the true results you are achieving.

Staying on the once-a-week schedule is a more accurate depiction of your progress. Any scale available at Walmart or Target will work fine, so don't feel like you have to break the bank on a fancy or high-tech one.

Bust Out the Tape
Because muscle weighs more than fat (and you gain muscle during exercise), you may not see all of your progress on the scale. Therefore, it is a good idea to take other measurements in addition to your weight to evaluate your achievements. Similar to the logic in weighing yourself on the scale, smaller measurements indicate progress. One of the most common measurements to take is your waist. The proper place to take a waist measurement is between the end of your bottom ribs and the top of your hip bones (usually right at your belly button). Use any soft measuring tape that will completely wrap around your waist. Other measurements you can take to monitor your weight loss progress include the circumferences of your thighs, hips, and bustline (mainly for females).

Body measurements are good markers of progress and encouragement, especially when the scale is not showing the success you feel you should be seeing.

Check the Tags

Everyone knows that when you are trying to lose weight, it's a good sign when your clothes become too big for you to wear. Pay close attention to the size printed on the tags in your clothes as they start and continue to become smaller. Don't hang onto those old, baggy clothes either. You have to have the mind-set that there is no turning back once you start to lose weight and live healthy. Therefore, don't ever think that you should keep your "big" clothes just in case—get rid of them!

Visual Progress

Perhaps the best way to track the progress of your weight loss journey is to look in the mirror. When you stand facing yourself in the mirror, can you tell that you have lost weight? Are you starting to feel better about your self-image? Are you starting to look like a different person after shedding pounds? Try taking pictures of yourself at different intervals (weeks, months) and look at the changes in your body.

Losing weight is about feeling better about your appearance.

If you are continually feeling more self-confident and proud of your appearance, then you are definitely making progress!

Reward Progress

Along with tracking the progress you make during your weight loss journey, reward yourself for accomplishing milestones along the way.

Set up intermittent goals during your weight loss journey and as you reach them, reward yourself with something you enjoy.

If you are trying to lose, say, fifty pounds, set small goals in between for every ten pounds you lose and treat yourself at those points. That way, you have different milestones along your journey for which you can be proud of and reward yourself accordingly. However, rewards should not be food related. This can stimulate your brain to associate success and achievement with certain foods and can cause a major setback in your weight loss journey.

You don't need to create another barrier to overcome, as everyday life creates enough already.

Instead, try rewarding yourself with something similar to the following:

- Workout apparel, shoes or accessories
- Electronic gadgets
- Spa visits
- Vacations
- Days off from work
- Books, movies or tickets to concerts

You've worked hard and you deserve to be rewarded for it!

Take a Vacation

If you are on a diet twenty-four hours a day, seven days a week, you are inevitably going to end up driving yourself crazy. Even if you're trying to lose weight, it's not against the law to treat yourself occasionally to something that you love to eat. The last thing you want to do is to become bored or frustrated with your diet and then suddenly throw it all away.

With that, it's important to allow yourself a "splurge" day every week to relax and rejuvenate your weight loss journey.

It's almost like a short "vacation" from your diet. Keep in mind that you should limit treating yourself to a single serving or meal (think moderation). Stay away from eating an entire half-gallon container of ice cream or visiting the all-you-can-eat Chinese buffet down the street. It's also best to take these short vacations from your diet after you have checked in to track your progress, and not right before. The last thing you want to do is discourage yourself in any way from what you have been able to accomplish thus far.

Establish a Support System
To successfully lose weight, it's important to surround yourself with people who will support your initiative and goals.

Significant Other Support
One of the most influential people in your life is your significant other.

The decisions that you and your significant other make directly affects the other person in some way, shape, or form.

It is important to get your significant other on board from the beginning as you start the path of losing weight. There are many ways that your husband, wife, life partner, boyfriend, or girlfriend can support you during this process, but perhaps the two most important ways are through positive reinforcement and assistance in avoiding temptations.

- **Positive reinforcement:**
Tell your significant other up front as you begin your journey that you need positive reinforcement along the way. He or she needs to tell you as often as possible that you are looking thinner, your clothes are looking a little loose, you are looking good in a bathing suit, or whatever makes you feel good about yourself. After all, this is someone who usually sees you every day, so they should be able to notice any progress you make.

- **Assistance in avoiding temptation:**
It makes it much more difficult to successfully lose weight when temptations to be "bad" surround you. Seek the help of your significant other not to bring unhealthy foods into the house and/or make suggestions for meals that are not

good for you. Also encourage them to engage in exercising activities with you. It will make it easier for you to get regular exercise done when you have someone willing to do it with you. You will also be less apt to stay home in front of the TV all evening if your spouse is not making that option available. It's not surprising, too, that often as someone starts to lose weight, his or her significant other does as well.

Friends and Family Support
If you do not have a significant other or if you want additional support, enlist the support of your closest friends and family members. Like a significant other, friends, coworkers, siblings, children, parents, and anyone else close to you can provide great support and assistance in helping you lose weight.

Support Groups
In addition to seeking support from the people closest to you, it often helps to have the encouragement of people seeking the same goals. Do a search online to find support groups near you. Some of these support groups are in

classroom and discussion settings, while others consist of weekly progress checks.

Finding something that keeps you motivated and in line is all that matters, regardless of the approach.

Rest

Your mind and body need ample rest and an opportunity to recharge. If you are not getting enough sleep, you are creating a huge speed bump on the road to achieving your weight loss goal. As humans, we need 7 to 9 hours of sleep every night according to the Centers for Disease Control and Prevention (CDC). Sleep helps your cognitive skills, enhances your mood during the day, strengthens your immune system, and keeps your heart and blood vessels in great shape.

If you don't get the needed amount of sleep, your body will crave salty and sweet foods.

This will, of course, not be a good catalyst to eating right and improving your dieting habits.

Additionally, not getting enough sleep will make you suffer from fatigue when exercising. Your body won't be well positioned to complete workouts, and you'll ultimately lose steam in making the effort to just show up at the gym. A lack of sleep, even more importantly, can over time increase your chances of developing heart disease and diabetes.

Prepare for Success

Losing weight and living healthy is just as much about your mind-set as it is your physical actions. You have to prepare mentally to be able to make significant changes in your life if you hope to succeed in the end. Make sure that you are thoroughly prepared to succeed before you start your weight loss journey!

- Define the reason and purpose to motivate you to achieve the results you're seeking
- Set goals so that you have a target you are aiming to reach
- Establish a method to track and reward your progress along the way
- Plan specific vacations to take from your diet and exercise routines

- Surround yourself with people who truly want you to succeed and will help change your life
- Get an appropriate amount of sleep each night to put your body and mind in an optimal position for success

**Keep It Simple and Elementary...
Eat Less, Exercise More!**

eat less

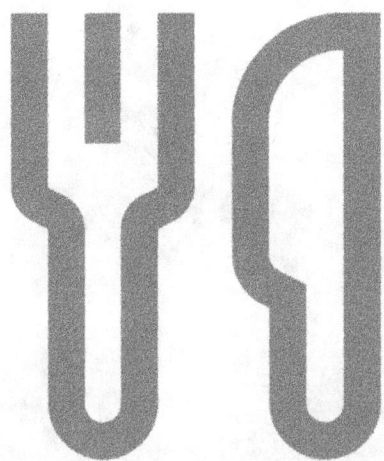

Eat Less

thoroughly enjoy spending time on my MacBook laptop, iPhone and iPad. Whether it's reading articles, checking out new apps, streaming media, shopping, or just mindlessly browsing the web, spending my free time across these devices is something I gravitate towards quite frequently. The web provides so many avenues of information, entertainment and resources that I don't see how we survived in the past without it. However, I know that as part of being an adult I have other responsibilities, obligations, and goals to tend to in my life, so I do my best to limit the amount of time I spend in front of these devices (excluding my work obligations).

The point here is that life is best enjoyed in moderation. You should never deprive yourself of things you enjoy and that make you happy. At the same time, however, too much of a good thing can definitely be, well, not very good at all. This is especially true with food. It's fine to treat yourself to something that tastes delicious, but it is also important not to overindulge.

Plan to Eat Well

Losing weight is not about starving yourself or excluding certain types of foods (e.g., limiting carbohydrate intake). To live a healthy life, you need a number of different nutrients from every food group. Each of these nutrients fuels your body to work properly and make you feel good.

The healthier your body is, the more receptive it will be to losing weight.

Here are some of the most important nutrients your body needs and what they do to help you.

- **Proteins:**
Numerous parts of your body are nourished by protein, including your bones, muscles, cartilage,

skin, and blood. Protein is your body's core building block.

- **Carbohydrates:**

Carbs are both your body and brain's main source of energy (especially during physical activity). A healthy level of carbohydrates is essential to ensure your body and mind are running at full capacity.

- **Vitamins and Minerals:**

Vitamins (such as A, B, C, D, and E) and minerals (such as calcium, iron, zinc, potassium, magnesium, and selenium) protect, restore, and fuel your body in a number of ways. They enable your bodily systems (nervous, cardiovascular, and digestive) to perform efficiently and aid in the formation of red blood cells to help your body fight off diseases and viruses. They also protect and maintain your skin, nails, eyes, hair, teeth, gums, and bones, and may even reduce high levels of blood pressure and bad cholesterol.

Types of Foods to Eat

Your everyday diet should encompass a variety of foods that are rich in the essential nutrients your body needs to make you feel your best and reach your WLG. Below are some healthy and common options to include in a balanced diet.

- **Proteins examples:**
  - o Extra-lean meats
  - o Skinless poultry
  - o Egg whites (or Egg Beaters)
  - o Beans
  - o Nuts and seeds
  - o Fish
  - o Fat-free or reduced-fat dairy
  - o Tofu

- **Carbohydrates examples:**
  - o Whole grains
  - o Fat-free or reduced-fat dairy
  - o Fruits
  - o Vegetables

- **Vitamins and Minerals examples:**
  - o Most foods contain vitamins and minerals. Different foods have varying compositions of vitamins and minerals, though, which means it's important to consume a wide variety of foods. Pay close attention to

nutrition labels to learn the vitamin and mineral content.

o Consuming a variety of fruits and vegetables is an easy way to take in numerous vitamins and minerals.

Grocery Shopping Essentials

In order to eat the foods that are essential to a healthy diet, you must first buy them. That's why weight loss and healthy living is directly correlated to the food you purchase at the grocery store.

If you buy a healthy variety of foods, you'll have a much better chance at losing weight.

If you buy unhealthy foods, you'll have a much tougher time shedding the pounds.

The following are some general guidelines to follow when making a trip to the grocery store.

- **Make one trip per week:**
  o Avoid making multiple trips to the store each week. Stick to one day a week to shop for all of your food.

- **Plan ahead of time:**
  - o Before you make the trip to the store, plan your meals for the week. This keeps you on task while shopping.
  - o Plan for your healthy snacks as well. Remember, Elementary Weight Loss is about being smart and sensible.

- **Make a list before you go and stick to it:**
  - o For the meals you have planned to eat each week, make a list of ingredients you will need. Stick to this list while in the store and don't deviate from it.
  - o Make sure the foods on your list include the essential nutrients you need.
  - o Avoid discounted items if they are not on your list—even though they may be very tempting to purchase.

- **Spend the majority of your time in the perimeter of the store—avoid the middle aisles:**
  - o The perimeter of most grocery stores contains more fresh and essential foods for your diet.
  - o Produce (fruits and vegetables), lean meats (fish and poultry), and dairy products are in

this area of the store and should be your focus.
- o Middle aisles in grocery stores usually contain junk food.
- o Although there are items you will need in the middle aisles, don't spend a lot of time browsing in this section (you might get yourself in trouble).

- **Focus on whole foods:**
  - o Select items containing 100% of the advertised item (e.g., 100% fruit juice or 100% whole grain).

- **Stay away from foods with a laundry list of ingredients:**
  - o The fewer ingredients a food item has, the more natural and likely more healthy it is for you because it will contain fewer artificial ingredients.

- **Make your visit after a meal (don't go hungry):**
  - o If you make your trip to the grocery store on an empty stomach, you are more likely to throw something in your cart that you wouldn't have purchased otherwise.

Eat Small, Eat Often

In addition to eating the right foods, the size and frequency of your meals is essential to losing weight.

Eating small meals frequently throughout the day is the key to successful dieting and weight loss.

Eat Smaller Meals

It's not only the types of food people eat but the sheer amount as well that makes it hard to lose weight. Stuffing yourself with a big meal is not conducive to a healthy lifestyle. The key to losing weight is learning to eat smaller quantities of food. Eating small meals can be difficult in the beginning because you are retraining your mind and body that a smaller amount of food can be just as satisfying. The good news is that it gets easier and easier with each smart decision you make to eat small.

Below are some tips to keep your meals the right size.

- **Don't let your stomach fool you:**
  - o Sometimes your stomach can make you perceive that you are hungrier than you actually are. Your stomach might fool you

into thinking you are "starving," which can lead to your eating much more than you should. Always trust your better judgment in these situations to make the smart decision to eat small. Are you really starving?

- **Use smaller plates:**
  - o Using a smaller plate, such as a salad plate, during a meal allows you to control the amount of food you serve yourself. Larger (entrée) plates have much more area on them to fill with additional food that you most likely don't need. The less room on the smaller plate means less food that you can fill it with. Do you really need a larger plate?

- **Avoid second helpings:**
  - o It's important to note that using a smaller plate doesn't give you the right to refill it. Multiple small plates are just as bad as one large plate. Stick with one plate during a given meal even if there is more than enough food. Can you live without a second helping?

- **Cut the "clean-plate" mentality:**
  - o Never feel like you have to eat everything on your plate during a meal—especially

when you don't have the option of using a smaller plate. Not eating every crumb of food is by no means against the law. Do you have to eat every last bite?

Eat More Often

Believe it or not, a key to losing weight is eating more frequently. Ingrained into our society is the fact that there are three meals a day—breakfast, lunch, and dinner. Three meals a day is well suited for your average skinny John Smith or Jane Doe. However, not everyone is blessed with an efficient and speedy metabolism (which is like a car engine in your body). There is hope, though, because like many other parts of your body, your metabolism can be trained to perform at a desired level.

The rate at which consumed food is burned and used as fuel in your body is highly dependent on your metabolism. Basically, eating fewer meals during the day will slow down your metabolism, whereas eating more meals will speed it up. This is because the longer your body has to wait for its next meal, the longer it will take to burn off the previous meal. Therefore, if you make your body wait several hours for more fuel, it will hold on to the fuel it has and burn it much slower to prevent your body from being without energy for long periods of time. However, the more often you eat, the faster your body thinks it needs to burn the energy from your last meal because it knows it will be getting more fuel in much less time. To put it simply:

Fewer Meals Each Day...
→ Results in a Slower Metabolism
→ Results in Gaining Weight

More Meals Each Day...
→ Results in a Faster Metabolism
→ Results in Losing Weight

- **The Six(2)Plan:**
  - o This is where the **Six(2)Plan** comes in. One of the best ways to speed up your metabolism is to eat six small meals a day—spacing out your meals as evenly as possible so that you can train your metabolism for maximum efficiency. Eating roughly every two hours throughout the day, starting with breakfast, should give you plenty of time to get in your six meals.

In case you haven't put it together yet, the Six in the Six(2)Plan represents the number of meals a day you should eat, and the (2) represents how often you should eat them (every two hours).

o The Six(2)Plan begins with a healthy breakfast. Breakfast is the most important meal of the day because it jump-starts your metabolism for the entire day. An example daily meal schedule might be organized similar to the following:

→ 9:00 a.m.—Breakfast 1
→ 11:00 a.m.—Breakfast 2
→ 1:00 p.m.—Lunch 1
→ 3:00 p.m.—Lunch 2
→ 5:00 p.m.—Dinner 1
→ 7:00 p.m.—Dinner 2

o Allow two to three hours after a meal before going to bed. Allowing time for your food to digest before heading off to bed will help your body process the food more efficiently because you are still moving around more frequently than if you were just lying in bed. It can also help to prevent indigestion. Indigestion can be uncomfortable and cause loss of sleep, which is not helpful in achieving your weight loss goal.

Staying Out of Trouble

Eating smaller portions and spreading out your meals throughout the day won't be easy at first. It will be hard to fight off late-night cravings and overeating at meals. Amazingly, though, your appetite will decrease over time as it gets used to the smaller meals. You won't want to have as much food and will get full quicker.

During times of temptation, look at your before picture and remember why you want to lose weight.

This will help keep you motivated and out of trouble. Trust me... it will get easier over time!

Below are some tips to get from one meal to the next without snacking and to cut out late-night urges.

- Chew sugar-free gum in between meals. Not only does it tide you over from one meal to the next, but it also keeps your breath smelling fresh.

- Brush your teeth as soon as you are done with your last meal of the day. Food never tastes the same right after you brush your teeth, and it is a way to mentally help you acknowledge you are done eating for the day.
- Stay active. Keeping busy and involved in nonfood-related activities gets your mind out of the snack zone. Most people snack purely because they are bored.
- Stay away from the kitchen. If you hang out in or near the kitchen, snacks are easily within your reach. Out of sight, out of mind!

Eat Out Intelligently

Planning to eat well at home is one thing, but planning to eat well while dining out is another ball game. You must make informed decisions of what and how much you eat when eating outside of your home (e.g., at a restaurant, fast-food establishment, social event, or another's residence).

Restaurant Rendezvous

Dining out with friends and family is an enjoyable experience that is a normal part of everyday life.

However, eating at restaurants can have a serious impact on your diet and weight loss journey if precautions are not taken.

The impact restaurant food can have on your diet stems from not only the ingredients in the food but also the sheer size of the servings.

Therefore, when you are eating at restaurants, you must make smart and healthy decisions, and be willing to ward off any temptations to eat poorly.

- **Order wisely:**
  - You don't have to be a genius to know that the rack of baby back ribs or the half-pound bacon cheeseburger with french fries is not as good for you as the grilled chicken plate with vegetables or the baked salmon entrée. Lighter fares such as sandwiches, soups, salads, grilled chicken, and grilled fish are usually the best bets.
  - If your meal comes with sides, substitute the normal greasy selection (fries or chips) for another item such as steamed vegetables,

fruit, beans, or a side salad. You can do this at most restaurants.

o If you order a salad, be aware of all the toppings included. Substitute crispy fried chicken with grilled chicken, and avoid other unhealthy items such as bacon. Select a fat-free or light dressing to go along with your salad, and ask for dressing on the side. It is better for you to have control over the amount of dressing used rather than the chef. Dipping each bite of salad in your side of dressing will also cut down on the amount used. Dressings are often the worst part of an unhealthy salad.

o If you order a sandwich, request that it be made on whole-grain bread or a whole-grain bun. Also request that the bread not be buttered. Many restaurants will butter or grease their breads for taste, which is obviously not healthy.

o Skip ordering appetizers or desserts, and stay away from the free basket of bread or chips on the table. An entrée is more than enough food for you to eat and usually contains more nutritious elements for your diet.

- **Think about quality, not quantity:**
  - Most people know that portion sizes at restaurants vary from place to place. Some restaurants serve more than enough food to stuff your belly, and others just barely satisfy your appetite. If the portion sizes are larger than the amount of food you should be consuming, then choose one of the following options (rather than abiding by the "clean-plate" mentality):
    - Share the entrée with someone else at your table. You can split the meal with a significant other, or just divide the remainder of your meal (after you have eaten your allotted amount) among friends and family.
    - Only eat what you should and save the rest for later. When you are served, immediately divide your meal into sections: one that you will eat at the table and the remainder that will be taken home as leftovers. Ask the waiter to put the take-home portion in a doggie bag so that you are not tempted with it sitting on the plate.

o See if the restaurant serves half portions. This will make it easier to eat only what you should. If you take your time eating, a smaller plate can turn into a more rewarding experience for your appetite. The slower you eat, the fuller you will feel at the conclusion of a meal. Eating slower also helps you enjoy the experience and your company even more.

- **Avoid overeating—even if the meal is free:**
  o For those who travel often for their jobs or are constantly entertaining clients with lavish meals, it is important to remember that just because your boss is picking up the tab, it does not give you a free pass to pig out. It's tempting when you are not covering the check to order a big, fat, juicy steak, or any number of unhealthy items you wouldn't normally splurge on. In situations in which your company, associates, or anyone else is paying for your meal, you must be strong and stick to eating the right foods in the right portion sizes. Check out the restaurant's menu on its website so that you can make a decision on your meal before you arrive at the restaurant. This

way, you won't need to browse the menu when you show up and be tempted by something you shouldn't eat.

- **Don't show up hungry:**
  - o The hungrier you are when you show up to a restaurant, the greater the chance that you will have a weak moment and cave in to temptation. Sometimes when we feel an extreme amount of hunger, we have a hard time saying no to types and amounts of foods we shouldn't eat. It's like a fight between your brain and stomach, usually ending with a KO (knockout) by the stomach. Abiding by the Six(2) Eating Plan should help alleviate this issue. However, if you still feel like you might be tempted by your current level of hunger before heading out to a meal, grab something small and healthy (e.g., a piece of fruit) just before leaving or drink a big glass of water.

- **Remove "all-you-can-eat" and "bottomless" from your vocabulary:**
  - o At the core of healthy restaurant dining is wisely choosing the restaurant. If possible,

stay away from places that offer all-you-can-eat or bottomless options; both are red flags. "All-you-can-eat" is a slogan many Americans live by, and more and more restaurants are offering bottomless menu items (as well as the free bread or chips you might receive before your meal comes). For more red flags and healthier alternatives, see the following FAsT-Food section (these apply to both fast-food and non-fast-food restaurants).

FAsT-Food

The fast-food industry is one of the largest contributors to the obesity epidemic and related health problems in our world.

There are minimal positive nutritional benefits and numerous negative health implications to eating most types of fast-food.

Most people already know this, yet they continue to support the fast-food industry. It's best to stay away from these establishments as much as possible.

If for some reason (although it's hard to think of any) you must stop at one of these types of establishments, make yourself aware of the following red flags and healthier options:

- **FAsT-Food red flags (stay far, far away):**
  o Special sauces—These sauces are usually loaded with mayo or sour cream, which means both calories and bad fats galore.
  o Cream-based sauces or soups—Some examples are chipotle, alfredo, mayo, ranch or blue cheese sauces, and any soup with cream in the name.
  o Smothered—This usually means at least twice the amount of cheese or a high-calorie sauce covering your meal.
  o Breaded or crispy—These words indicate the item is fried, and usually the breading cannot be removed from the meat.
  o Loaded—Loaded foods are topped with butter, sour cream, cheese, or other high-fat and high-calorie ingredients.
  o Blackened—This may seem like a better option, but it is a myth! Blackened meats are almost equivalent to fried meats because of the amount of oil that is used to create the seasoning.

- o Anything with cheese as the main ingredient—Examples include double cheese pizzas, cheese enchiladas, cheese-only ravioli, or quesadillas. Full-fat cheeses, which are high in calories, are typically used in fast-food establishments.
- o Supreme—A supreme dish is usually loaded with high-fat meats and/or other high-fat ingredients (e.g., sour cream and guacamole).
- o Biggie or super size—Larger portions can have two to three times the number of calories as a small or medium size.

- **FAsT-Food healthier options (an alternative if needed):**
  - o Go for the grill—Choose grilled dishes rather than fried or blackened options.
  - o Lean proteins—Choose items such as skinless chicken, turkey, fish, tofu, black beans, or veggie burgers, which are all good alternatives to beef and other red meats.
  - o Sauces and dressing on the side—Ask for all sauces and dressings on the side in order to regulate how much you consume.
  - o Stay with safe sauces—Sauces such as mustard, ketchup, balsamic vinegar,

Tabasco, salsa, and lemon or lime juice contain very low amounts of fat and calories and are great choices to make your food more flavorful.

o Lunch or kid-size portions—If you are allowed, choose the smallest portion possible to avoid overeating (you don't always have to be a child to order these menu options).

o Forgo the fries—Substitute veggies, fruits, beans, or another more healthy side item. It's well worth it even if you have to pay a bit more.

o Add more veggies—Veggies (raw or steamed) are almost always healthy options as toppings or side dishes.

o Wonderful whole- grains—Some restaurants offer whole-grain buns, rolls, pasta, and rice as alternatives, which fill you up faster and provide more fiber and protein.

o Do diet drinks or water—Substitute high-calorie, high-sugar beverages (including regular sodas, some juices, sweetened teas, punch, and lemonade) with a beverage that has little to no calories (such as diet soda, iced tea without sugar, and of course, water).

Surviving Social Events
At social gatherings, hosts tend to prepare much more food than will be eaten. This is so they don't look like cheapskates or appear rude for not being able to treat their guests. There is also the stigma that the hosts want their food to taste very good.

More unhealthy ingredients are typically used at social events because they are thought to create the best-tasting food (even though healthy ingredients can taste just as delicious).

The often plethora of food that is available and the type of food that is served are the two main reasons you need to be careful.

You might not want to seem like a recluse by not attending these types of events, so instead of making up excuses for why you can't go, try these alternatives:

- Let the host or hostess know ahead of time about your diet so they understand why you might eat less or decide to skip on some of the more unhealthy items served. The host or hostess might also offer to prepare a healthier dish that agrees with your diet.

- If it's a potluck event, contribute a healthy dish. In the worst-case scenario, you can just eat the food you prepared.
- If you are at a company party or similar event, make your food selections wisely and limit the amount you eat.
- Stay social. The more you talk and socialize, the less you will focus on eating.

Drink in Moderation

Whether it's out on the town or in the comfort of another's home, avoiding alcohol is a challenging task. Drinking is a social event often shared among friends, family, and acquaintances. Alcohol can be detrimental to your weight loss journey, as an average twelve-ounce bottle of light beer and an average five-ounce glass of dry wine each contains about one hundred calories. Keep in mind that figure is for light beers and dry wines—full-flavored beers and sweet wines can have more than twice as many calories per serving!

If you are more inclined to skip beer and wine in favor of hard liquor, be aware that the higher the proof the more calories consumed. Mixed drinks and fruity cocktails (such as margaritas and daiquiris) are loaded with sugar and hence calories.

You don't have to completely avoid alcohol when trying to lose weight, but rather, minimize its consumption and make smart choices when you do have a drink.

That means drinking a light beer or mixing hard liquor with a diet or low-calorie mixer. You might even skip the mixer altogether.

Brown-Bagging

Although it is possible to eat out and not sabotage your weight loss journey, it is still important to eat at home as much as you can. Try to make eating out a treat rather than a usual occurrence. Eating at home allows you to know exactly what you are putting in your body and is almost always more healthy than eating out. Taking food from home (i.e., a brown-bag meal) is also an easy way to avoid eating out when you are on the go.

If you bring your own food to work or school, then you won't be tempted to grab a sack of food from a drive-through during the day.

This strategy is also helpful in avoiding fast-food on road trips. Just pack a cooler full of premade meals to eat along the way. As a bonus, you also save money!

Drink Water

A healthy lifestyle and successful weight loss journey are both results of hydrating your body. That is why it is important to drink a lot of water throughout the day.

> **Water is plentiful, virtually free, and great for your health.**

Drink as much as you can each day to keep your body hydrated and to help you lose weight.

Why is Water Good for You, Anyway?

There are a number of reasons why water is good for your body and an essential component of a healthy lifestyle.

- **Water is plentiful and natural:**
  - o Why else would it cover so much of the earth if we were not meant to utilize it as humans?

- **Water is cheap:**
  o The cost of water coming out of the kitchen faucet or refrigerator door is negligible, and you can buy bottled water for a low price per bottle if you buy in bulk at a warehouse store or big-box retailer.

- **Water doesn't have anything bad in it:**
  o Pure water doesn't contain any calories, carbohydrates, fat, or sodium.

- **Water is the chief component of your body:**
  o Nearly every system in your body depends on water. This includes regulating your body temperature, lubricating your joints, protecting your organs, moistening your tissues (mouth, eyes, and nose), and flushing waste products from your body. Roughly two-thirds (60 to 70 percent) of your body is made up of water.

- **Water is a natural beauty product:**
  o An elevated level of hydration in your skin cells can make you look more vigorous and alive (rather than dull and dried out).

Drink, Drink, Drink It Up

Every time you breathe, sweat, or go to the bathroom, your body loses water. In order for the systems in your body to run properly, you must replenish your water supply. According to the Institute of Medicine and the Mayo Clinic, total daily consumption of water should be as follows:

- 13 cups (3.0 liters, or 100 ounces) for the average male.
- 9 cups (2.2 liters, or 75 ounces) for the average female.

One thing that those recommendations do not incorporate is the extra water that you will need to consume when you exercise. During exercise you sweat, which releases excess water from your body. The more you sweat during exercise, the more water you will need in addition to the recommended daily consumption. Because exercising is a big part of losing weight, as you will read later on, you need to consume more than enough water each day.

Proper hydration also gives you more energy, making exercise a little easier.

Many healthy foods such as fruits and vegetables contain a significant amount of water in them as well, and can be an additional source of replenishment throughout your day. Here are some easy ways to make sure you get enough water each day:

- Have water with each meal. Even if you are having coffee, juice, or a diet drink with a meal, have a glass of water next to your plate as well.
- Take water with you in the car. Many of us spend a lot of time driving to and from work each day. Take advantage of this time by drinking water.
- Keep water at your desk at work or school.
- Take water with you when you exercise.
- Keep a glass of water by you while you watch TV at night.
- Order water when eating out. It's free and you can take in a couple of large glasses during a nice leisurely meal.
- Keep a water bottle with you throughout the day and constantly refill it.

Eat Less

Losing weight and living healthy is not only about eating smaller quantities of food—it is also about eating less of the "bad" stuff. It's important to fuel your body with what it needs to function properly while at the same time not overindulging in any one meal or type of food—think moderation. Make a habit of eating less and eating well!

- Plan what you are going to eat in advance of meals by taking into account the right foods to eat—be a smart shopper.
- Don't just eat small meals. Eat them frequently throughout the day to train your metabolism following a methodology such as the Six(2)Plan.
- Make intelligent decisions when you are not the chef and are eating outside of your own home.
- Hydrate your body by drinking water all the time.

**Keep It Simple and Elementary...
Eat Less, Exercise More!**

exercise more

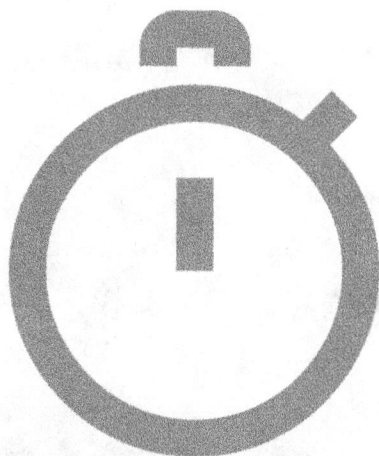

Exercise More

I have a natural inclination toward physical activity. I was an athlete across many sports growing up and as previously mentioned, a scholarship track and field athlete in college for four years. However, if you saw me at my current weight level, you would probably have a hard time guessing that I was a very large and hefty shot putter on the track and field team (as opposed to a sprinter). During college, my workouts consisted of not only lifting heavy weights in the gym, but also regularly consuming one-pound cheeseburgers and milkshakes at Fuddruckers to keep my body weight at a certain level.

When I graduated from college, I knew that I needed to make some major changes in my exercise routine to lose the extra weight. The treadmill became my best friend, and through hard work and determination (along with, of course, a revamped diet) I was able to lose 85 pounds, or about one-third of my body weight. The changes I made to my eating habits largely contributed to my weight loss success, but exercise was—and is—just as much a key component.

Exercise is a Must

Exercise is essential to any healthy lifestyle and successful weight loss plan. It's important to make exercise a high priority in your life. The act of exercising should be on the same level as eating, drinking, and sleeping—all life-sustaining activities.

The Benefits of Exercise

There are numerous benefits to exercising besides just burning calories and reducing your body's fat content.

Regular exercise makes you feel better, increases your confidence and self-esteem, helps prevent deadly diseases (including

heart disease, diabetes, depression, and certain types of cancer), and helps reduce stress.

These are all great reasons to incorporate exercise into your life! Here are some additional benefits of exercising:

- Reduces risk of high blood pressure
- Lowers bad (LDL) cholesterol levels
- Increases good (HDL) cholesterol levels
- Increases your energy
- Improves the functioning of your immune system
- Strengthens your heart and lungs allowing more efficient circulation of your blood
- Allows you to more easily participate in and perform everyday activities
- Improves your balance and coordination
- Slows the aging process in regard to some of the ailments that are linked to getting older (may help you to live longer)
- Increases your self-confidence
- Strengthens your bones, ligaments, and tendons (may reduce some chronic pains and prevent other injuries)

- Raises your metabolism so that you burn calories faster when your body is at rest
- Helps you sleep better at night

Active Exercise

Active exercise is when you make a conscious effort to participate in physical activity. This includes going to a gym, jogging around the neighborhood, or playing an active sport (one that makes you move around a lot such as basketball, football, soccer, or tennis).

You should participate in active exercise three to five days a week.

However, the more you actively exercise the better.

Cardio (Aerobic) Exercise

Cardio, or aerobic, exercise increases your heart rate and enables your cardiovascular system to function properly. It is an essential part of losing weight and maintaining a healthy lifestyle. During a cardio workout, you burn calories, lower your body fat content, and strengthen your heart and lungs. Types of cardio exercises or activities include walking, running, and swimming, among many others.

You should perform cardio activities three to five days a week for a minimum of thirty minutes.

Remember that active exercise means you are making a physical and conscious effort to work out for more than just a couple brief moments. Therefore, walking from the couch to the fridge is not considered active exercise!

Below are some types of cardio exercises along with brief guidelines and explanations. They're grouped into three categories: Unstructured Exercises, Organized Sports, and Structured Classes. Different activities are geared toward different levels of physical health, so please consult your physician before trying any exercise.

- **Unstructured Exercises:**
These are activities that are usually performed on your own, with a partner, or in a small group. They are referred to as "unstructured" due to your individual freedom in choosing the location, pace, time, distance, and so forth.

In your neighborhood, at a gym, at a park, or at the local high school track are just some of the many places you can perform unstructured exercises. Examples include:

- o Walking—Performed outdoors or on a treadmill. Keep up a brisk pace and use your arms.
- o Stair climbing—Performed using actual stairs or a stair-climbing machine.
- o Jogging—Performed outdoors or on a treadmill. Try implementing a walk/jog workout during which you rotate the two exercises.
- o Elliptical workout—Performed on an elliptical machine that simulates a jogging motion with less stress on your joints, bones, and tendons.
- o Running (sprinting)—Mainly performed outdoors. Try to keep distances shorter than one hundred meters (with multiple repetitions).
- o Swimming—Many different types of strokes can be used for swimming laps in a pool (butterfly, breast, side, back, etc.).
- o Bicycling—Performed on a standard bicycle outdoors or a stationary bike indoors.

- **Organized Sports:**

Some organized sports require you to be part of a team, while others allow you to compete on your own. Either way, these activities provide a good workout. Sign up for one of numerous recreational leagues and events in your local area, or simply compete with a group of friends at a neighborhood park. Examples include:

  o Football, basketball, and soccer—These are some of the most common team sports that will give you a good workout. However, just throwing or kicking the ball back and forth or shooting a few jump shots is not considered exercise.

  o Tennis, racquetball, and golf—These are individual sports that can give you a good workout. In order for golf to be considered exercise, you must walk the course and carry your own clubs. If you use a cart or a caddy, then you are not getting a good workout.

- **Structured Classes:**

Structured classes involve some of the unstructured activities mentioned above as well as many more. The great thing about taking structured exercise classes is that you usually have an enthusiastic leader or instructor and a number of other people doing the workout with you. This helps increase your motivation and performance levels. Many gyms and other stand-alone facilities offer an array of classes. Structured classes are usually more exciting than other forms of exercise due to the incorporation of music and high energy levels. They are also good for people who have a hard time being consistent with exercise. You usually meet people in classes who look forward to working out with you, and when you're not there, they will notice! Therefore, structured classes are a good way to hold you accountable to exercising on a regular basis. Examples include:

- o Aerobics—These classes combine a number of different movements and exercises into a single session. They take on many different forms including, but not limited to, step aerobics, water aerobics, and dance aerobics.
- o Spinning—Spinning classes are intense bike-riding sessions in a group atmosphere. They are performed on specially designed stationary bicycles.

o Kickboxing—These classes provide a total body workout and work nearly all the major muscle groups—including muscles you never knew you had!

You can search online for local recreational leagues, gyms, fitness centers, or individual facilities that offer any of the classes or athletic activities mentioned above. Don't be afraid to keep trying different exercises until you find ones that you enjoy and work well for you. Remember to start off at a slower, easier pace with any cardio (aerobic) exercise (one that matches your physical health and age) and then gradually build up over time. Increase the level, pace, and intensity just slightly each time you exercise, making sure you reach a point at which your heart rate increases and you can feel yourself getting a workout. There is no need to drive yourself to a point of exhaustion, but if you want to see your desired results, you need to "feel the burn."

Pumping Iron (Strength Training)
Contrary to what you might think, lifting weights (strength training) is just as important in the weight loss process as cardio exercise. You might be thinking, "I just want to lose weight... I don't

care about being big and buff!" The truth is that lifting weights is at the root of many of the benefits of exercising and has a direct correlation to losing weight.

One important benefit that strength training provides is increasing the speed of your metabolism.

This means that you burn more calories when your body is at a state of rest (e.g., when you are sleeping, watching a movie, or sitting in the car). The more lean muscle you have, which is acquired through lifting weights, the faster your metabolism becomes.

As you age, it's part of the human life cycle that your muscle mass naturally decreases. Another significant benefit of strength training is that it helps you fight the natural process of muscle loss. Otherwise, the lost muscle is simply turned into stored fat. Overall, "pumping iron" will allow you to look better, feel better, and be able to more easily perform everyday activities regardless of your age.

Don't worry if you feel clueless regarding how to perform different lifting exercises. The best thing you can do is to watch other people do them and pay attention to the illustrated instructions posted on many of the machines. Don't be afraid to ask for help. Most experienced lifters are eager to show off what they know. A number of gyms also offer free personal training sessions upon enrollment, so make sure to take advantage of those.

Strength training workouts should be completed two or three days a week for roughly thirty minutes.

Avoid lifting on consecutive days so that your muscles have ample time to recover (they need at least twenty-four hours).

- **Areas of focus:**
There are three main parts of your body to which you should tailor your weightlifting workout:

  o Upper body—Consists of everything above your abdominals. Major muscle groups include (with accompanying exercises):
    - Chest (bench press, push-ups)
    - Arms (bicep curls, tricep extensions)
    - Shoulders (shoulder press, lateral raises)
    - Upper Back (lateral pull-downs, pull-ups)

o Lower body—Consists of the area below the waistline. Major muscle groups include (with accompanying exercises):
  - Thighs and Rear End (lunges, squats)
  - Calves (calf raises)
o Core—This is the midsection of your body. Major muscle groups include (with accompanying exercises):
  - Abdominals (crunches, leg lifts)
  - Lower back (hyperextensions, bent-over rows)

- **Workout routines:**
In regard to a weight-lifting routine, the terms **reps** and **sets** are of utmost importance. Reps, or repetitions, are the actual number of times you perform the exercise motion. A set is a group of continuous and consecutive reps. For example, three sets of fifteen reps means you performed an exercise motion fifteen times at three different intervals (or a total of forty-five times). At each workout session, it is important to perform various exercises (I suggest six different exercises in a single workout session) that alternate between different bodily areas of focus and muscle groups, resting during and between each one. Here are

some guidelines to follow during a basic workout with six total exercises:

o Start with an upper body exercise, then move to your lower body, and finally to your core. Repeat this cycle twice working a different set of muscles during the second time through.

o For each exercise do three sets of fifteen reps. Rest thirty seconds between each set and two minutes between each exercise.

- **Amount of weight to use:**
How much weight you should use depends on your current physical shape and age. The only way to really find the right weight for you is through trial and error starting with a really light weight level and working up from there. You will have reached the appropriate amount of weight for an exercise when the last repetition you perform (the fifteenth rep) is challenging but not impossible to complete.

Stretch It Out (Flexibility)
One aspect of exercising that many people ignore is stretching. Stretching is extremely important to

your workout routine and should not be skipped or rushed through. First and foremost, stretching prevents injuries by warming up your muscles and keeping your joints flexible.

If you work out without stretching your muscles, you are more susceptible to becoming injured.

Injuries hinder exercise and can significantly slow down your weight loss plan. In addition to keeping you flexible and preventing injuries, stretching can help promote better posture, relieve stress by relaxing tight muscles, and promote more attractive looking muscles.

- **What to stretch:**
You should concentrate on your major muscle groups (those discussed in the Pumping Iron section—upper body, lower body, and core) when stretching. Here are some guidelines for a basic stretching routine (feel free to perform additional stretching exercises if needed):

  o Perform three or four upper body stretches, three or four lower body stretches, and three or four core stretches.

o Hold each stretching exercise at a point where you "feel the stretch" (holding point) without any pain for fifteen seconds.

- **When to stretch:**
Stretching is not an activity that should be performed only once during a workout (i.e., before you start). Rather, you should stretch at the beginning and end of an exercise session, as well as at times when your body is sore when not exercising:

o Stretch before—Stretch at the start of (or before) each workout. Spend a couple of minutes prior to stretching warming up your body with low-intensity movements (walking, jogging, jumping in place, etc.). Stretching cold muscles before a workout can be even worse than not stretching at all, which is why your body needs to be warmed up first.

o Stretch some more—Stretch at the conclusion of your workout. The after-workout stretching session is the most beneficial because your muscles are fully warm at that point.

o Stretch when sore—Stretch when your body is sore from working out. It will make you feel a lot better, improve your flexibility, and make it easier to remain consistent and continue working out during this uncomfortable period.

Have Fun and Mix It Up

Working out doesn't have to be like pulling teeth. Try to find something you enjoy doing.

Making exercise enjoyable will allow you to stay consistent and see the results you desire.

Keep in mind that different exercises work different parts of your body, so it's important to mix up the types of exercise you do.

Making Time

A lot of people say that they don't have time to exercise, but that is a poor excuse. No matter what you or anyone says, there is always time in your day to exercise. Whether it is early in the morning, at lunch, in the evening, or even late at night, you should always be able to incorporate exercise into your life. You have twenty-four hours in any given day, and active exercise only has to take up about one of them. It shouldn't be too hard to figure out that *you really do have time.*

Passive Exercise

Passive exercise is physical activity incorporated into your daily routine, rather than a predetermined "workout" that you have scheduled time for. This includes doing things around the house, at work, at school, or wherever else you spend your time during the day. Some common examples are taking the stairs instead of the elevator and parking at the back of a parking lot so that you have a longer walk to your destination.

Passive exercise can make a significant difference in your weight loss.

However, keep in mind that passive exercise is a *supplement* to active exercise, not a substitute for it.

"Fit" It In

There are many areas of your life in which you can incorporate exercise without going to a gym or anywhere else you would actively exercise. Whether you're at work, at home, running errands, or even out on the town, there are always numerous opportunities to get in passive exercise. As previously mentioned, passive exercise is supplemental to the active exercise you are already doing. Passive and active exercise work hand in hand. As you perform active exercise consistently and lose weight, passive exercise activities will become easier and more commonplace (vice versa as well). Everyone has different schedules and performs different activities throughout each day, and it's up to you to figure out how to fit in passive exercise. Examples of passive exercises you can do throughout the day include the following:

- **Take the stairs instead of the elevator or escalator:**
  - o This applies to anywhere (within reason) that gives you the option to climb stairs.
  - o If you have stairs in your house, make excuses to use them as much as possible. If you live in an apartment or condo, do the same with the community stairs in the building.

- **Park in the parking spot farthest from entrances:**
  - o Park at a distance that will maximize how far you have to walk to your destination. Avoid the temptation to find the "perfect spot" near an entrance.
  - o When making a quick trip to the shopping mall, park at the opposite side of the mall from your desired store.

- **Regularly perform chores around the house (don't pay someone else to do them):**
  - o Set aside a couple of days each week to perform both outside (mowing the lawn, tending to plants/flowers, etc.) and inside (dusting, mopping, sweeping, etc.) chores.

- **Instead of sitting when you are waiting somewhere (e.g., doctor's office, dentist's office, hair salon, airport), get up and walk around:**
  - o Purposely show up early to an appointment, the airport, or any other place where you might wait so that you can spend some time walking around while waiting.

- **Take advantage of any time you can lift or carry something:**
  - o Carry your own grocery or shopping bags when running errands.
  - o Carry your luggage while traveling instead of rolling it.

- **Enjoy life to its fullest:**
  - o Dance, sing, smile, laugh, clap, cheer, and—by golly—hug someone! Having fun and being happy always gets you moving around.
  - o Play with your kids (or borrow someone else's if you don't have any). Participate in activities with children that cause you to get up and move around.
  - o Try something new or engage in hobbies you like to do (snorkeling, hunting, gardening, sailing, etc.).

WOW (Working Out at Work)

Doing small things at your place of work to increase physical activity and making sure you are not just sitting on your

bottom all day is what WOW (Working Out at Work) is all about.

For many people, work consists of sitting on your rear behind a desk for at least eight hours a day. During this time you most likely have zero physical activity and burn little to nil calories or fat. This can greatly hinder your objective of losing weight if you don't make the best of it. After all, if you are going to spend the majority of your day working, why not take the opportunity to lose weight while doing it?

Below are a number of things you can do throughout the day that will help to minimize the time you spend sedentary at your desk. Even if you don't spend all day in a typical office environment (lucky you) or if you are a stay-at-home parent, you can still incorporate many of these activities into your schedule.

- Physically get up and talk to others when you need something. Don't just stay at your desk to call or email people.
- Keep your meals in the community break room so that you have to get up and walk to get them. Avoid keeping meals at your desk.

- Spend part of your lunch break walking around. It doesn't take you a full hour (if you have one) to eat, so use what extra time you have left to get in some activity.
- Use the stairs whenever possible and make constant excuses to do so.
- Don't worry about getting the best spot in the office parking lot. Park in the back and walk.
- Stand up while on the phone or computer if possible. There are even desks designed for you to be able to stand up while working.
- When you drink lots of water throughout the day, you will have to go to the bathroom more often. More trips to the restroom equals more walking.
- Alternate using your water bottle every day with a small cup one or two days each week. This will cause you to have to get up often to refill it.
- Try not to sit in your chair any longer than thirty minutes at a time. Get up and walk around at least twice every hour.

Exercise More

Losing weight and living healthy is a product of not just dieting, but just as important, exercising.

Exercise is essential to successful weight loss and provides numerous other benefits that can enable you to live a long, healthy life. Make sure exercise is a part of your everyday routine!

- Actively exercise by participating in scheduled workouts that incorporate aerobic, strength training, and flexibility components.
- Passively exercise through everyday activities, including making the best of the time you spend at the office.

**Keep It Simple and Elementary...
Eat Less, Exercise More!**

Live A Healthy Life

Like anyone who has lost a sizeable amount of weight, I was very proud of myself after dropping 85 pounds and becoming a much healthier person. It is definitely one of my biggest accomplishments in life. However, I am even more proud that I have continued to keep the weight off and live a healthy lifestyle. Losing the large amount of weight was just the start of it all!

Just the Beginning
After losing weight and hopefully reaching your WLG, it's easy to think that the hard part is over. Well, I have news for you… the hard part is just about to begin!

Just because you lost weight and are now living a healthy lifestyle doesn't mean that you can do a 180-degree turn and go back to frequent fast-food meals and a sedentary lifestyle.

You have to keep that weight off and continue to live healthy.

You have worked too hard to turn back now! After all, looking better, feeling better, and being healthier is what you put all that hard work in for anyway, isn't it?

The After Picture

Take an **after picture** of yourself after you've reached your goal. You probably are much more excited about being in front of the camera now and will surely be taking many more pictures. Remember the before picture you used along your journey as motivation? Grab that photo and keep both the before and after pictures in the same place going forward. They can be in a side-by-side frame, in a photo album, sitting in a drawer together, or anywhere else you'd like. The photo comparison is going to be a major source of motivation not to put the pounds back on. If you ever feel an urge to get back into the bad habits you worked so hard to break, pull out these pictures and look at them side by side. Focus on how you looked and felt back then in the before picture and how you look and feel after reaching your WLG in the after picture.

Elementary Lifestyle

What you've been through is a transformation rather than just a temporary deviation from your old lifestyle. You should still follow the principles of Elementary Weight Loss going forward. Remember, Elementary Weight Loss is a lifelong change, not just a quick fix.

- Your accomplishment is now your motivation to stay healthy and keep off the weight. Don't forget what it feels like to feel the way you do now.
- Continue to track your weight and measurements, and reward yourself for maintaining your current healthy lifestyle.
- Get enough sleep and give your body the appropriate rest it needs.

- Eat healthy foods and keep your diet balanced. Take in all the appropriate nutrients your body needs and thrives on.
- Make smart choices when grocery shopping and stick with a system that has worked for you. Continue to plan to eat well.
- Moderation is still essential. Use portion control at mealtime and eat more frequently than the traditional three meals a day—remember the Six(2)Plan. Make sure that breakfast stays in your eating schedule and don't skip meals during the day.
- Make smart decisions when you eat out at any other venue besides your own home—especially at restaurants.
- Never stop drinking water.
- Exercising is still—and always—a must. Don't stop now!
- Continue to make active workouts a regular part of your weekly schedule.
- Keep up the things you've been doing as passive exercise, as they should be commonplace and a normal part of your life now.

**Keep It Simple and Elementary...
Eat Less, Exercise More!**

Weight Loss Resources and Tools

Y̶ou can find a current list of weight loss resources and tools online at **www.elementaryweightloss.com/resources.** In addition to a number of websites and apps, you will find tools to help guide you throughout your weight loss journey.

Furthermore, below are some online resources affiliated with Elementary Weight Loss that will help you with preparing to lose weight, eating less, and exercising more.

Snapweight

- Find it online at **www.snapweight.com**.

Snapweight provides simple and effective motivation to lose weight. With Snapweight, you can utilize the tools and influencers within your social networks to help motivate you to lose weight.

Six(2)Plan

- Find it online at **www.six2plan.com**.

Six(2)Plan provides a simple way to speed up your metabolism. With Six(2)Plan, you can find easy meal recommendations to follow a schedule of six small meals every two hours each day that train your metabolism for maximum efficiency.

Calendarfit

- Find it online at **www.calendarfit.com.**

CalendarFit provides workouts that are made specifically for your calendar. With CalendarFit, you can reach your exercise and fitness goals by easily adding workouts to your calendar with simple and convenient exercises you can do anywhere.

THE END

Good luck losing weight and living
a healthy life!

**Keep It Simple and Elementary...
Eat Less, Exercise More!**